CHRISTIAN SCIENCE, MEDICINE, AND OCCULTISM

A CRITICAL WORK

First Edition 1902
Albert Moll M.D.

New Edition 2019
Edited by Tarl Warwick

COPYRIGHT AND DISCLAIMER

FOREWORD

This little booklet is one of a number of manuscripts made by the famous Albert Moll, and is predominantly critical of occultism. I provide it here (despite being an occultist myself) as a stark warning to other practitioners- like Moll, it is best to seek first to rationalize and, what is left unexplained, is the real diamond in the rough to investigate further. In this way the occult is fundamentally not dissimilar from science, and where a mundane explanation exists, supernatural ones are of relatively lower import.

Here, Moll does not actually discredit the concept of faith healing being useless, but rather insists that its successes (which he points out are not numerous- which is indeed true today as well) are due to mesmeric ability. In the modern sense, we relegate the successes to a perhaps different rung of reality and invoke the neural with the placebo affect. He suggests, though, that at least in some instances Christian Science may be of use- in the modern era, it is fairly well established (even spoken of openly by accredited professors and doctors) that for many complaints- which are ultimately stress or mind related and not purely otherwise physical) any placebo- prayer, a sugar pill, etc- will do.

This edition of "Christian Science, Medicine, and Occultism" has been carefully edited for format and content. Care has been taken to retain all original intent and meaning.

CHRISTIAN SCIENCE, MEDICINE, AND OCCULTISM

When I was traveling in 1898 for some months in the United States of North America for the purpose of making a general survey of the country and its civilization, the principal question, besides the hackneyed phrase, "What do you think of America?" put to me was, "What is your opinion of Christian Science?" In New York, in San Francisco, in Boston, in Denver, in Chicago, in New Orleans- everywhere the same query. Before leaving Europe I had, of course, heard and read about Christian Science; but I was astounded to find the doctrines of this creed spread over the United States to an extent which is scarcely suspected on this side of the ocean. Upon my return here I was frequently asked by my colleagues, as also by laymen, about the scientific conditions of America. I often warned my questioners not to depreciate the progress of science in the United States, and incidentally gave vent to my opinion that ere long we should have to combat a new psychical epidemic emanating from America- viz.; Christian Science. Past events show that such epidemics generally follow along the highways of commerce; yet a psychical epidemic with a tardy beginning, but attaining a high pitch of development, spreads rapidly and takes deep root; in fact, it would be well-nigh miraculous if in this instance an exception were to be recorded.

Of course, I was often met by the rejoinder: "We shall never fall a prey to so palpable a swindle; it is merely American humbug!" But to the practiced eye, following impartially the trend of civilization in the United States, where not only industry and commerce flourish in an uncommon degree, but where science as well is pursued with unbounded enthusiasm, the mere mention of such words as "'American,' humbug," and 'swindle' in the same breath appear as a delusion. America is no more the land of humbug and swindle than are the States of the Old World. After all, so far as psychical epidemics are concerned, what does it matter whether the intellectual standard of one country is slightly superior to that of another? The susceptibility for psychical epidemics is in no way affected thereby; the difference between civilized countries is too slight, but the similarities are very pronounced. Psychical epidemics naturally find the same fertile ground for development in Germany as in the United States or in England, or any other country, since all nations consider themselves the most enlightened, and look upon others with a certain disdain.

Who does not remember, in Germany, for instance, the commotion created even in the highest circles of cultured society by the spiritualistic medium, Slade? Where was table-turning more in vogue? When a few years ago a Mrs. Abbott, the 'Magnetic Lady,' by the clever application of the laws of leverage, and with the necessary *sang-froid*, demonstrated on the stage her 'magnetic powers,' by which she defied the combined resistance of several men, it was considered the height of conceit and presumption to make reference to the scientific doctrines of leverage and to deny the existence of magnetic powers.

Again, so far as disease is concerned, what a vast amount of abuse has not been practiced with the voltacross in bodily ailments of all sorts. The shepherd quack Ast could boast in his days of a bigger clientele in Germany than the most notorious American charlatan ever had at home. As for Berlin, we need not go back to the olden times, when towards the end of the eighteenth century the cult of the mystic arts held high revel. Much is said of the acumen and intelligence which is to be found in Berlin. So far as that is concerned, it may suffice to quote here Perty's remarks on a certain occasion in 1849. The rush to see the 'Infant Prodigy,' Louise Braun, was so great that pickets and police patrols were necessary to keep the crowds in order. Dr. Mielay, who was entrusted with the examination of the case, was chagrined at the gullibility of the inhabitants, who, whilst sneering at the sacred tunic of Treves, allowed themselves to be duped by a girl scarcely thirteen years of age.

Still more recently, who does not remember the Schweninger craze, which swept over Berlin about fifteen years ago, affecting many people even of the best classes of society? I protest, however, that in saying this I have not the slightest intention of casting a slur upon the personality of Dr. Schweninger. Nevertheless, thousands of people suddenly believed that to find a cure for their divers affections all they had to do was to abstain from drink whilst eating, and to observe the many other regulations laid down for the so-called Schweninger cure.

Again, when, a few years ago, Goolam Kader, yclept 'Indian oculist,' came to Berlin, his house was literally ill besieged by patients hailing from every class of society. Susceptibility for psychical epidemics exists, therefore, in Berlin as well as throughout Germany and elsewhere. Under these circumstances, the vigilant mind is not surprised at the sudden excrescence of Christian Science among us, and we find that as spirit-rapping penetrated from America to the Old World, so has Christian Science also found its way across the briny deep.

What is the origin of this Christian-Scientistic or metaphysical method of healing? The founder of it is a Mrs. Eddy. She is said to be now about eighty six years of age, and has thrice been married. She first entered wedlock in 1843; her third marriage took place in 1877, when she was of the tender age of sixty-one. The third husband, I am told, was an old pupil of hers. She has been a widow since 1882. Even in Scientist circles her third marriage gave offense, as it was looked upon as something a trifle too worldly. Mrs. Eddy originally devoted herself to the practice of homoeopathy, and is credited with having discovered her new method of treatment in this pursuit, or rather, as some assert, through an accident which befell her in 1866. She suddenly recovered from a severe internal injury after reading a certain promise in the Gospel, although she had been given up by her medical attendants. Mrs. Eddy began to practice her metaphysical faith-cures at Lynn (Massachusetts), and went from there to Boston, where she established, in 1881, the Metaphysical College, and trained many pupils. She lives now in Concord (New Hampshire), but has retired from practice. Of the twelve works which are accredited to her, the best known is 'Science and Health: Key to the Scriptures.' What an enormous circulation this book has attained may be judged from the fact that the first copyright was taken out in 1875 in Washington, and after twenty three years- i.e. in 1898- had reached its 145th edition. In 1899 alone thirty new editions were issued, thus making 175 editions in twenty-four years.

The movement reached Germany through a Miss Schoen, a native of the Rhenish provinces- her father was a civil servant- who for several years acted as a teacher of the German language and literature at the State University in Minneapolis. (Miss Schoen lays particular stress upon this fact as a proof that she is a lady of culture. For the benefit of those who are not so well acquainted with the conditions prevailing in America, I may mention that the rank and standing of Universities in the United States vary considerably. Several of these Universities are, no doubt, the peers of the best of similar European institutions, but the State University of Minneapolis cannot be reckoned among these.)

The first central station was established in Hanover. Here a sister of Miss Schoen joined her, and the two worked together with a Mrs. Dr. Gunther. About a year and a half ago a central station was established in Berlin, which is presided over by one of the Misses Schoen, but the other sister frequently makes visitations. There are other central stations in Germany- viz., one in Hamburg, in charge of a Miss Neumann; another in Breslau, under a Miss Vette. Other central stations in Germany are not recognized by the Misses Schoen as genuine.

Of course, Christian Science is practiced in many German towns and cities. Quite recently a Mrs. Seal came from America, and settled down in Berlin to practice faith-cure. She made overtures to Miss Schoen for amalgamation, but without success. Miss Schoen's advice was to confine her practice to the American element residing in Berlin. No doubt she could be of great use to them, but, as she was unacquainted with the German language and required an interpreter, her usefulness among the natives must necessarily be impaired, as it is indispensable for successful operation that healer and patient should be in complete rapport. Miss Schoen assumes the national standpoint; "Germans for the German; Americans for the American." Even though we assume that Miss Schoen's opinion is based on good faith, there are two objections to it. First, it is not quite clear why the healer should be required to possess a perfect knowledge of his patient's language, since, as we shall see later on, but few words suffice for the treatment.

Besides, treatment may be administered even from a distance, and children, imbeciles, lunatics, and animals are not excluded from the faith-cure. The second point which deserves mention is, that the Christian Scientist evidently is afraid of the same competition which makes itself felt in all other pursuits of life. A characteristic feature is that one faith-healer often warns his patients against other faith-healers, and advises them to beware of those who only claim to be healers, but have in reality no control over magnetic powers. One distrusts the other, exactly as one quack claims the quality of healing for himself alone, but disputes the claims of all the others. But, perhaps. Miss Schoen has no material interest, after all, in disclaiming her relationship to her colleague ; maybe her action is solely prompted by injured vanity, since Mrs. Seal adopts the same method of treatment without having first obtained a diploma from Miss Schoen. Besides these, I am told that several other nurseries of Christian Scientism have recently sprung up in the German realm- for instance, one in Stettin, where, according to newspaper advertisements, a preacher and his wife practice the faith-cure. However, it is a fact that those healers who cannot trace the origin of their knowledge to Mrs. Eddy are not acknowledged as of equal rank by the Scientists.

Now, what does really happen at these so-called faith-cures, or healing by prayer? To start with, these expressions are quite incorrect, for there is no treatment by faith or prayer. From time immemorial prayer has often been employed for healing purposes. A few years ago a charlatan, S__, was sent to prison. His cures always commenced with prayer, which began early in the day and generally lasted till 10:30. Prayer-books were not required for the purpose, as he had his own original prayers, such as, 'All pain ceaseth, if God pleaseth'; then came a foot-bath, or something similar, followed by prayer till sunset. For this performance S__ received from each of his patients eight shillings, and from the police magistrate one month.

Towards the end of the eighteenth century a certain Chevalier de Barbarin created a big sensation in Ostend. He produced magnetic sleep, but it was necessary that he should keep vigil with prayer by the bedside of his patient. But ordinary prayers such as the aforesaid are not the routine employed by the Christian Scientists. Take the case of Miss X__ (the patients are generally ladies). Upon her arrival at Miss Shoen's establishment, the following takes place: "Please, madam, take this chair. It is quite immaterial whether you sit down by the window or the stove; only concentrate your thoughts upon this one point: My illness is the outcome of sin. God does not desire sin. God will cure me. I place my trust in Him alone." The patient being seated, Miss Schoen settles down in another chair, and begins to concentrate her thoughts hard on the same point, viz., that God will cure the patient. Prayer does not take place, only a concentration of thought on the same subject. At times an explanation of the treatment is given to such as ask for it; for instance, that the illness is not the work of God, for God sends neither disease nor sin. The patient is cautioned not to think that her illness is the consequence of her own sins; rather is it the cumulative sequence of the sins of mankind in general. Stress is laid upon the relation that exists between mind and matter, particular reference being made to Berkeley's philosophical system of subjective idealism, according to which matter is defined merely as an imaginary quantity. Separate treatment is given to each individual case, and endures, according to circumstances, from a few minutes to a whole hour. It is repeated according to success. Some patients are treated daily, then at longer intervals, whilst others start on the long periods at once.

The question why two persons are necessary for this faith-cure is met by the answer that the mind of one person exercises its influence upon that of the other; that this power is not given to all, as it is found in some in a higher, in others in a lower degree, whilst the majority of people cannot influence others at all.

As has been indicated above, there is also a treatment from a distance. For instance, Miss B in H writes: "Require three days' treatment for distressing muscular pain in right hip." The case refers to a lady who, whilst lifting up a child, experienced a sudden stitch in the back. A swelling in the hip ensued, which of course disappeared forthwith upon sending the telegram to Miss Schoen. F. B in P telegraphs: "Please give immediate treatment for internal injury." This is followed by a letter giving details. The sender had received a blow which broke a rib and affected the lower lobe of the lung. Soon after sending the telegram at 9 p.m. relief is experienced. Miss Schoen tells me, however, that treatment from a distance is of quite exceptional occurrence. Yet in the published reports this healing from a distance plays a very prominent part. All possible ailments are treated from a distance, even diphtheria in children. Treatment from a distance is extended to persons even quite unknown to the healer, and is indicated when the person is unable to travel. This, however, is claimed to happen but rarely. It is more successful by far where a certain rapport exists already between the patient and the healer, a sort of a 'current' between the two persons, as it were. If a former patient of Miss Schoen's should happen during a sojourn in Italy, for instance, to feel a sudden attack of pain, it suffices to acquaint Miss Schoen of the fact by telegram.

The hour for treatment and concentration of thought is arranged by wire, and the cure is accomplished. I have already spoken of currents which work from a distance, and are said to be very effective in this treatment. Faith in Christian Science on the part of the patient, although very desirable, is, however, not a condition *sine qua non*, as good results may be obtained without it if the surroundings are favorable. A cure is much more easily effected when the parents, brothers and sisters, relatives and friends, of the patient have faith in Christian Science, for in this wise many currents are concentrated upon the sufferer and produce a favorable issue. This principle is of importance in the treatment of children, imbeciles, and lunatics, who cannot concentrate in the required manner. In children especially the best results are recorded. It is often simply astounding how quickly children show reaction. When they attain the age of seven or eight, and know something of God, perfect miracles are wrought on them as soon as they are instilled with an absolute reliance in the Lord.

Smaller children, who know nothing as yet of God, require the assistance of their parents. In the case of demented persons, who cannot enter into rapport, the necessary faith must be supplied by others. These are never treated at the establishment, as the surroundings there are unfavorable for the necessary conditions. Animals, too, it may be mentioned here, are influenced in a like manner. The faith of others plays an important part in the treatment of man as well as beast, but not only the faith of those in the immediate surroundings, but also that of those in nowise connected with the sufferer. Its significance will be plainly understood from the following words taken from Mrs, Eddy's principal book: "When a patient dies from a dose of poison against the expectations of doctor, patient and relatives, death may be thus explained. Although in such an event a few persons may have the belief that the stuff taken is harmless, yet the great majority of mankind, though ignorant of this special case, believe that, e.g., arsenic, strychnine, etc., are poisons. It follows that the final result is influenced by the outside majority, and not by the small minority in the sick-room. In other words, Mrs. Eddy is of the opinion- If someone dies of strychnine in spite of his belief that he will recover, his death is due to the circumstance that the majority of people assume strychnine to be a deadly poison; that is to say, the opinion of the majority constitutes a poison to be deadly or otherwise.

And yet a book which contains such absurdities is put by the Scientists on a par with the Bible!

The next question here is: What ailments, which diseases, may be cured? The sweeping answer is: All! Hysteria, nervous disorders, gastric fever, affections of the throat, nose, and ear, cancer, internal injuries- it makes no difference. Only in one case the Christian Scientist admits that outside assistance is required. It won't work for broken bones! And yet in this instance it would be appropriate to say: "*Hie Rhodus, hie salta!*" For here, indeed, the injury is right under one's fingers, under one's nose! Why should faith in God be insufficient in such cases? The Christian Scientist admits that in this emergency the injured part must first be bandaged and put in splints according to the rules of surgery; i.e, an interference must be effected by that well-hated school of the medical arts. The insufficiency of Christian Science is thus explained. The fracture must be reduced and the injured part made immovable, as otherwise the patient might spontaneously move, and thus arrest the process of healing. But this is a fundamental error, for the movements which are observed in fractures are by no means spontaneous. On the contrary, the sufferer is only too happy when he need not move the injured limb.

It is the involuntary contractions of the muscles that shift the broken ends of the bone and make splints necessary. The objection of spontaneous movements will not do. It is admitted that not all patients are healed, although all diseases are healable. Particular care should also be bestowed upon patients who have been taking physic for some time, and in consequence are run down. The use of physic in such cases ought not to be suddenly stopped, as the point should be carefully weighed whether this might not have a deleterious effect, as in many systems the tissues would be too much worn away by drugs to be restored by the mind. But even in such cases symptomatic advantages can be achieved in so far as troublesome conditions will show improvement; e.g. in cancer, pain will be removed even though death were not forestalled. In other cases experiments must first be made as to the possible influence of Christian Science upon the disease, thus necessitating, as it were, a period of probation.

Definite promises of success are never made. Miss Schoen herself, as well as her patients, admits so much. As to the question of diagnosis, we are told that such is never made. It is contrary to the principles of Christian Science, which looks upon sin as the cause of disease, and the belief in God as the only remedy for it.

When a diagnosis is asked for, the patient is told: "You must consult a medical man on that head. We do not object if you wish to find out what your ailment is; neither do we mind if you prefer to place yourself under medical observation; but the treatment must be confined to our own methods. Medicines must under no consideration be administered. Persons who show anxiety we always persuade to be first examined by a doctor, not because we believe that a medical man could benefit the patient, but because exaggerated fear and nervousness are obstacles to the efficiency of our treatment. A short time ago a lady came to us suffering from various complaints. She was much worried, and evidently anticipated cancer. We persuaded her to be examined by a medical man, and told her that, even though he should diagnose cancer, she must by all means come back to us, as we would undertake the cure. Well, the doctor laughed at the idea of cancer, and we soon relieved her of all her ailments."

Payment is another very interesting point. In Berlin you pay 3 marks for every sitting, no matter how long that may last. In Hanover local customs are considered, and the tariff is accordingly lowered to 2 marks. No charge is made to the poor; nevertheless,. the fact remains, as Miss Schoen naively remarks, that all patients prefer to pay something. If treatment extends over a long period, the charges are on a reduced scale, and those whose means are limited meet with every consideration. "The reduced tariff is always suggested by us; but we are often told that it is not wanted. In fact, a higher remuneration is frequently offered, and not seldom even forced upon us, although we have never accepted more than 3 marks in Berlin, and 2 marks in Hanover."

Of course, so far as payment is concerned, I do not take

the exalted position that to earn money is a disgrace; nor is it a contradistinction to the *bona-fides* of treatment by Christian Science if money is paid and accepted for it. Meetings are frequently held in the evenings, at which instructive lectures on Christian Science are given, Mrs. Eddy's book being used as the foundation. Spiritual songs form part of the ceremony. But these meetings are not used for the purposes of propaganda, as the audience consists chiefly of patients. This, however, is not quite correct, for admission is open to all comers.

Occasionally the history of a specially interesting case is given. Treatment, cure and prayer are not practiced at these meetings, which are rather looked upon as preparatory exercises, to point out the fundamental principles of Christian Science, viz., that sin is the root of all disease, and that the latter can only be healed by the influence of mind over matter. In spite of all this, cures are frequently chronicled at these assemblies. Twice a year- i.e., in the spring and in the autumn, regular courses are given, each lasting from eight to ten weeks. Three meetings of two hours' duration are held daily. The subscription to these courses is 400 marks. Less than that amount cannot be accepted, since a regulation was made by Mrs. Eddy that a universal charge of 100 dollars must be made all over the world.

In France they pay 500 francs, accordingly. However, modifications are made- not that the price is reduced in any way, but payment is accepted on the installment plan, especially from such as are training for the office of healer. The latter is really the main object of these courses. The pupils must give full proof that they possess the psychical element which qualifies for the position of healer. The novices must undergo a term of training covering a period of not less than six months, during which time they must frequent the Central Depot under the immediate management of the Misses Schoen. Extra-metropolitan pupils must reside for four weeks in Berlin before they can be admitted to the Institute, thus giving an opportunity for inquiry into their character.

As a rule, not more than eight or ten pupils are admitted, though on one occasion there were as many as fifteen applications, but only five were favorably entertained. The knowledge of English is a very important factor, as Mrs. Eddy's books are only written in this language. The followers of Christian Science claim that their healing methods are based upon the Bible; of course, it is easy to find references in the Bible to certain relations existing between sin and disease. In my book on 'Medical Ethics,' recently published, the following passage will be found in corroboration of this assertion: "In several places does the Old Testament refer to sin as the cause of disease. Woman is threatened with dire bodily affliction should she become guilty of adultery. Other instances are the Black Plague of Egypt, the pestilence among the Israelites in the days of King David, the withered hand of Jeroboam, the leprosy of Gehazi, the illness of Hezekiah. Similar observations may be found also in the New Testament; e.g., Christ ascribes the thirty-eight years' suffering of the paralytic to the sins of his youth."

Nevertheless, it cannot be said that the theologians have at all times looked upon disease as the natural sequel to sin. Diedrich, whilst quoting in his 'Doctrines on Christian Morality' examples of sin being the cause of disease, contends that such a connection could not be traced in all cases, though perhaps in many. Of the beggar blind from his birth and healed by Christ, it is said that neither he nor his parents were guilty of sin; in fact, "he was born blind that the works of God be made manifest in him." The Book of Job is another proof that in the Old Testament, also, disease was not always considered as a punishment of sin. At any rate, the Christian Scientists have no ground for deducing from the Bible a general relationship between disease and sin. Of course, all sorts of relations exist between disease and religion. Remember Lourdes and other shrines to which pilgrimages are made by the halt and ailing to find relief and cure. Attention may be called here to the care and nursing of the sick, the development of which art reflects immortal praise and merit upon the Catholic Church. Again, why are public prayers offered up to the Almighty the world over for the recovery of eminent sufferers? On the other hand, neither the Bible nor the Christian religion will support the fundamental contention of Christian Scientists, that matter exists only in the abstract- a principle to which, by the way, they themselves frequently stand in opposition.

I will not enter here upon a discussion as to whether Christian Scientism contradicts the Bible. Its followers deny it; the theologians assert that it does. At any rate, the opposition of the Church to Christian Science is quite palpable, and, from her standpoint, justifiable, because the adherents to Christian Science are formed into a new sect, and have adopted their own religious service. In Hanover, for instance, quite a number of people have left the Established Church to join the new religious movement, which, however, has not yet assumed the same proportions as in the United States, where, for instance, in Chicago the Christian Scientists possess already four churches. The ecclesiastical authorities act, consequently, quite within their right when they preach against Christian Science, even though many of those who have affiliated with the latter still remain, to all appearances, active members of their former churches. Christian Science, indeed, glories in the fact that its blessings are bestowed on all religions. And it may be freely admitted that in other directions most of the Scientists are quite free from prejudice. For instance, they are strong advocates of cremation, since "matter is something of little importance- in fact, does not exist- and the mind cannot be affected or destroyed by fire."

The object of this treatise, however, is to discuss the

relation of Christian Science to medicine rather than to theology and religion. Medicine absolutely ignores the question whether sin is the cause of disease; it rather busies itself with the pathological changes that may be observed in the nature of man, and looks upon illness and disease as disturbances in the anatomical conditions and functions of the body. This standpoint must be always taken by the practitioner in the choice of his remedies. Being an applied natural science, medicine must needs adhere methodologically to the tenet that effects are the results of certain causes; that, so long as effects can be explained as the results of certain causes, no other explanation is required. Only when this explanation proves an utter failure should new and unknown forces be looked for. This principle must govern the administration of every medicine. If we apply it to Christian Science, the question naturally arises:

What opinion can we, as professional men, form of the alleged faith-cures? Is it necessary here to assume that certain mystic, psychical forces are transmitted from the healer to the patient? Is the alleged cure in reality an effect of the thought that disease is the natural outcome of sin; that God does neither wish sin nor disease; and that faith is all-sufficient for the removal of disease?

The answer is decidedly, No! For the results claimed by Christian Science can, without the aid of obscure or mystic powers, be explained by well-known natural forces. Much has been said and written of late years of suggestion. In fact, this has become a kind of generic term for all sorts of things, and includes many complicated psychic processes. Suggestion, however, comprehends by no means everything that comes here under observation. Suggestion really means the production of a desired state by awakening the conviction of its existence. If you tell a person who easily blushes, "Why, how red you are growing!" that person will certainly blush. This is a suggestion.

CHRISTIAN SCIENCE, MEDICINE, AND OCCULTISM

Suggestions of this kind frequently suffice to remove pathological symptoms; in other words, the awakened conviction of their non-existence causes the symptoms to disappear. Hypnosis, which enhances susceptibility considerably, is a great aid to suggestion, although in many cases it may well be dispensed with. The faith of a patient in a remedy prescribed acts as a suggestion. Thus, the principles of suggestion may often explain the faith-cures produced in many persons who believe in Christian Science, as they are firmly convinced that this particular treatment will benefit them. But in Christian Science other motives come under consideration, not the least of them being emotion, which plays a prominent part in the conditions of man. At Lourdes, for instance, not only is suggestion a significant item, but also, the enormous excitement produced by the surroundings is a predominant factor. The same takes place in the treatment by Christian Science, where the existing effects of anticipation are of no small moment. The anticipation of coming events is the father of divers sensations.

According to Carpenter, anticipation may produce functional changes in the human system, even without the aid of direct suggestion. It is self-evident that in susceptible persons who believe in Christian Science an exaggerated state of anticipation predominates. Just imagine the emotions of a person sitting down and agitated by the all-absorbing concentrated thought, "What is coming next?"

Another point must not be lost sight of, viz., to divert one's thoughts is often sufficient to render one oblivious to symptoms- for instance, pain, at least for the time. It is impossible in a short essay like this to analyze all the various psychical processes. But one thing is certain; that if, under ordinary circumstances, psychical influences offer advantages in the treatment of disease, it is quite unnecessary to resort to Christian Science for that purpose, or, in other words, to engage the sudden and direct intervention of Mrs. Eddy or her emissaries between God and the patient. All the cases where a cure or improvement was claimed, and which I had the opportunity of seeing and testing personally, were only disorders of a functional character, such as hysteria, nervous debility, etc.

Functional diseases in medical parlance are those in which no organic changes take place. Even granted that there is no disease in which organic changes do not take place in one form or another, in functional affections these changes are so imperceptible that hitherto they have been considered a negligible quantity. Yet even among functional diseases there are some in which organic changes are supposed to exist, although the nature of such changes is as yet unknown to science in its present stage- e.g., palsy. In others these changes are of a transient character. An hysterical woman has a headache today; tomorrow she feels a twitching in the arm ; the day after she is quite lame, or, on the slightest provocation, she has spasms.

Although these indications may point to a collapse of the nervous system, yet the organic changes which form the substratum of the pathological symptoms are not of such a permanent character as to warrant an explanation of these sudden symptomatic variations. But these cases of hysteria, of general nervous debility, and of rheumatic affections, offer a remunerative field for the exploits of psychical treatment. Undoubtedly in the treatment of many of these ailments Christian Science can boast of unqualified success.

Neither will I dispute that Christian Science is capable of improving the symptoms even when serious anatomical changes are present; but that is no reason why we should look upon it as a direct intervention of God at the bidding of the Christian Scientist, for in ordinary psycho-therapy, especially with the aid of suggestion, the same results are obtained. I will not discuss here the question in how far organic changes may be furthered by psychical influences, and in how far these influences may also affect pathological organic changes, but for the explanation of psychical reactions in organic diseases the following may suffice. We will admit that enduring psychical influences cannot be considered without organic changes taking trace. For instance, the constant pursuit of a certain avocation delineates characteristic features on the physiognomy- to wit, the typical face of the clergyman. Neither can we deny that even transient psychical influences may, under circumstances, leave behind them unmistakable traces on the body. Anguish, fear, fright, terror, relax the muscles of the urinary and rectal plexus, bring on premature parturition, etc.

If a suggestion be made to a person in the hypnotic state, that a blister has been put on a certain spot of the skin, anatomical changes may often manifest themselves in that particular spot. Notwithstanding these observations, I do not believe that psycho-therapy can lay claim to any influence when the removal of anatomical changes is considered. And if now and again we hear of marvelous achievements in this direction, we are still justified in accepting such reports with a large measure of diffidence. But psychical influences may also operate in other directions where anatomical changes, and even organic disorders, are concerned, and thus produce, particularly in the mind of the lay person, an illusory cure. In this regard the following points must not be lost sight of: First of all, in anatomical diseases the functional disturbances frequently affect a wider area than corresponds with the real focus of the attack. In cases of paralysis, for instance, the primary disturbances are much severer than those observed after the lapse of a few days or weeks.

In some cases the anatomical lesion spreads considerably, and yet the functional disturbances, such as paralytic inhibitions, relax, and even disappear; but this does not justify the assumption that the anatomical lesion has been healed. As has been said before, the functional disturbance often covers a wider area than its anatomical center seems to justify. Probably this is due to the fact that under the influence of the anatomical lesion other parts of the nervous system have received a shock which produces a functional disturbance, and we may, therefore, assume that the parts thus inhibited will in due time recover functional powers. Moreover, other organs, or parts thereof, frequently undertake, for the time being, the functions of the organs affected.

Now, with regard to the treatment of organic diseases, it is a well-known fact that ordinary psychotherapy, especially suggestion, is successfully applied for the removal of disturbances of a merely functional character; and the assumption that God, at the special request of the Christian Scientist, has suddenly intervened is quite gratuitous. In fact, the assertion that God would, because the Christian Scientist is concentrating her thoughts, vouchsafe to suddenly cure her patient is rather a blasphemy than an acknowledgment of the inscrutable works of the Almighty. The Christian Scientists claim that by their method, not only are the symptoms improved, but the disease itself is cured, even if, in the opinion of the medical expert, such a disease, according to well-established experience, must prove fatal unless the skilled physician or surgeon interferes- e,g, cancer or spinal affections. I remember a case of suppuration of the spinal cord in a girl, which, it is claimed, yielded to faith-cure.

Other cases are quoted in which surgical operations were advised or even performed without the desired result, but which were miraculously cured by the application of Christian Science. These cases may be divided into two groups. To the first group belong those cases in which an operation was really performed without success, but in which, at any rate, a marked improvement was observed when taken in hand by Christian Science. Much as I should like to concede even this, yet I cannot accept the claim without a challenge. I am convinced that every neurologist- nay, every experienced physician- has had in his own practice to deal with patients who, after having been treated locally, or even operated upon by some specialist for this or the other complaint without success, showed at once favorable reaction when subjected to the proper psychical treatment. Specialists frequently become one-sided in their views, and are too prone to seek the cause for pathological symptoms in an affection of that organ of which they make a specialty. Thus, often enough the otologist erroneously attributes pains in the head to an affection of the nasal organs, confounding an abnormal condition with a disease. But this simply deals with the excrescences of specialism, which the practical physician soon recognizes, and uses as aids to modify his own opinions. As a matter of fact, a strong undercurrent of opposition has made itself felt of late in professional circles against the excessive mania for operations and local treatment. It is sincerely to be hoped a daring diagnosis like this could hardly be based on medical authority, and may well be looked upon with suspicion.

That this movement will eventually succeed in repressing specialism, and re-establishing the general practitioner in that position to which he has a well-founded claim. The surgeon and, in many instances, the specialist are ever too ready to operate, because their opinions are biased, and they erroneously attribute nervous symptoms to some organic derangement. How often, for instance, has castration in cases of hysteria proved a dismal failure, whilst methodical psychical treatment soon brought the desired relief. For the same reason, a woman who has been unsuccessfully treated for some time by a gynecologist may find under Christian Science speedy improvement, if not complete restoration. In these cases the simple question arises, "What sort of treatment is likely to impress the patient most deeply?" And if this happens to be that by Christian Science, we surely have no right to dispute the latter's claim! Nevertheless, even that cannot force us to admit that the will of God is at all times at the disposal of the Christian Scientist. We can only perceive in it the psychical effect, especially suggestion.

The second group comprises incurable diseases such as cancer, etc., which Christian Science claims to have cured. The first question arising here is: "Who made the diagnosis?" Was it made by a trustworthy medical authority or not? We must know his name and his standing. It is not sufficient that the patient herself should aver, "A doctor told me I had cancer." Such a statement is too vague, and does not deserve credence. There are many people in the world who consider it a great distinction if they can boast that once upon a time they suffered from an incurable disease, and were, in fact, given up by the doctor. In my own practice I have been told by patients that their own doctor had given them up, whilst I found the very opposite to be the case when reference was made to that doctor. There are persons who seem to derive a ghastly pleasure from the thought that they have already been standing with one foot in the grave. Before we are asked, therefore, to believe these tales of wondrous cures, let us have the name of the man who diagnosed cancer, etc. The reports of the Christian Scientists seem to, dearly prove that the diagnosis in these instances was generally made by themselves, and that no medical authority was consulted. But whether this can satisfy the demands of science, of which the Scientists brag so much, must remain a matter of very grave doubt.

An American doctor has offered a premium of 1,000 dollars to anyone who can prove that in a single instance through the instrumentality of Christian Science a congenital malformation has been corrected. Another medical man has proposed to inject a lethal dose of poison into a follower of Christian Science to see it counteracted by faith-cure. Till now no one seems to have accepted these challenges. So far as the latter proposition is concerned, it may be remarked here that successful experiments have been made with castor-oil when the subject was placed under the influence of hypnotic suggestion without the aid of Christian Science.

A person is given a dose of castor-oil sufficiently large to produce the natural effect. The hypnotic suggestion that the effect shall not take place until forty-eight hours have elapsed is successfully made. It is therefore apparent that with the aid of suggestion much can be accomplished which at first sight may seem impossible. Hence it becomes necessary to first eliminate all sources of fault before the theories of Christian Science can be adopted as established facts. Moreover, in many cases a spontaneous improvement of pathological symptoms may take place without connecting its cause with any given method of treatment.

As a characteristic case in view may be quoted a miraculous cure said to have been effected by the notorious Russian priest Johann on a paralyzed woman when consecrating a new church. The woman simply became overexcited and fainted, and recovered from her spell as soon as the priest put in an appearance; but there is no evidence whatever to show that the recovery was in any way due to the influence of his presence. But, argues the Scientist, why is it that we have no failures to record? For Christian Science has treated many persons who have suffered not only from functional and not necessarily fatal diseases, but also from affections which the recognized school of medicine classifies as incurable, and yet failures are unknown to us. My reply is: In America frequent untoward results are reported- to wit, the many actions for damages brought in the law courts against Mrs. Eddy and her disciples. Whether a true verdict has ever been found or not, I do not pretend to say. If not, it only proves that according to American law a conviction cannot be obtained. Even in this country such would probably be the case if the healer adopted the necessary means of precaution. If proper precautions are taken, no ground will be left to the patient upon which to base a charge that he was in any way restricted from consulting a physician, or prohibited from undergoing the regular medical treatment, or that its course was improperly influenced. In America, even convictions in offenses against industrial legislation are difficult to obtain, because freedom of trade does not exist there.

Although there are today only three States in the Union in which an official diploma for the practice of medicine is not required, yet in all the States the legislatures have enacted special laws exempting those who heal without the aid of medicaments. Such persons do not come under the head of medical practitioners. But the principal point here is that failures in Christian Science- and there are many of them indeed- never find the light of publicity. Those chiefly concerned do not care for exposing themselves to the ridicule of their fellow creatures, for people who have been taken in, as a rule, do not like to admit it. There are plenty of people who have turned to Christian Science for help, but, failing to find the desired relief, stoutly deny that they ever went there, and certainly do not boast of their futile attempts.

No one likes to own that he was made a fool of. That is precisely the reason why the majority of cases of swindle and crime committed by confidence men, blackmailers, gamblers, and the like, never come to the knowledge of the police authorities. The victims prefer suffering the loss to exposing themselves and their stupidity to public derision. The next point to consider is. What relations- if any- exist between Christian

CHRISTIAN SCIENCE, MEDICINE, AND OCCULTISM

Science and occultism? For the benefit of those who are not sufficiently acquainted with the meaning and bearing of this point, I will briefly elucidate the subject by a few examples: Two persons, X and Y, are making the following experiment: X is in one room of the house, Y in the other. Y is told: "Here is a piece of paper and a lead pencil; X will fix his thoughts upon a certain number. As soon as you become conscious of a certain fixed number, write it down on this slip of paper." X now thinks intently of the number 93, and Y writes down 93 on his slip of paper. In occultism this transference of thought from one person to another without perceptible interference of the senses is commonly called telepathy, or mental suggestion, and it is claimed that in this manner, under given conditions, will, thought, even sensations, may be transferred from one person to another, even from a great distance.

A yet farther-reaching field for occultism is the doctrine of animal magnetism by which it is assumed that A exercises a special influence over B by means of animal magnetism-suggestion is excluded. This special power is, however, to be found only in privileged persons. So far as the effect itself is concerned, the contention is that A can by means of animal magnetism cure diseases in B; that A by magnetizing B can make the latter impervious to pain; that A can also produce in B peculiar conditions which cannot be explained in the ordinary way; that by A's magnetism a somnambulistic condition is established in B which brings to light certain faculties foreign to him in his normal, or demagnetized, state. For instance, a dislocation of the senses is claimed to take place such as will enable B to read with the pit of his stomach or some other part of the anatomy. Still further, it elicits the faculty of clairvoyance of space and of time; thus, B is enabled whilst in London to discern things that happen in Paris (clairvoyance of space), or to foresee things which will happen in the remote future (clairvoyance of time.)

CHRISTIAN SCIENCE, MEDICINE, AND OCCULTISM

But there are numerous other manifestations part and parcel of occultism. Spiritualism is a favorite hunting ground for the occultist. This, again, may be subdivided into two groups, viz., spiritism in the narrower sense and psychism. Both have in common the doctrine that at times manifestations become apparent which cannot be explained by the ordinary laws of Nature. The commonest phenomenon is spirit-rapping.

Mysterious noises are heard in tables, or other pieces of furniture, or in the walls; furniture is moved about in an unaccountable manner without mechanical interference. To this class belong also the so-called rapports from an invisible world. In Berlin quite recently a Mrs. Rothe- the noted flower-medium- created a sensation. She made innumerable flowers appear, and distributed them among the faithful as gifts from the spirit world. Apparitions of the spirits of the dead were conjured up, and the spirits themselves were made visible to the mortal eye. All this, of course, was attributed to the influence of the medium, and claimed to be beyond the powers of the ordinary person; but one day a police detective exposed the wily tricks of the clever dame, and put an abrupt end to the fraud.

The spiritualists are divided into two groups. The spiritist, in the narrower sense of the word, believes that the spirits of another world produce strange phenomena, such as table-rappings, pulling those present by the beard, and similar jokes. All this is commonly thought to be the work of the spirits of the dead. Some, however, assume that certain spirits dwell among us common human beings, who, because indiscernible to the material eye, make themselves known to us in this strange manner.

In opposition to this spiritualistic creed, the psychists, on their part, contend that these peculiar phenomena observed at times are not attributable to the direct interference of spirits, but are rather the result of mysterious psychical powers, possessed and exercised by so-called media. In this wise manifestations such as table-moving, closet-rapping, etc., are accounted for. Christian Science is a near relative to occultism; in fact, it is only a branch of the latter. Proof of this may be found in the query: "What is the homogeneous factor of all manifestations in occultism?" About five years ago Dr. Ferdinand Maack made an attempt to arrive at a definition of occultism by sending out a round-robin to all the experts on the subject known to him. The circular was also addressed to me, and my answer was that two conditions are necessary to qualify a claim to occultism- first, that either the phenomenon itself, or the cause producing the phenomenon, or the relations existing between the cause and the phenomenon, are foreign to our general knowledge. If, for instance, a fakir is buried for months without access to food and to air except through the pores of the ground or the coffin in which his body is confined, and he yet survives, this is a phenomenon not universally recognized as a possible fact.

Serious doubts exist in the mind of the scientist whether the body of the fakir really ever entered the coffin. Thus it happened a few years ago that two fakirs, who were traveling through Europe with the object of demonstrating the possibility of this feat, were on a certain occasion, a few days after they had been to all appearances interred, arrested in a cafe whilst enjoying a game of cards. And yet at the same time a watch committee, who had been appointed to see that the two individuals did not leave their confinement or partake of food, were still in faithful attendance at the coffins.

When pieces of furniture suddenly begin without perceptible mechanical cause to move about a room, the occultist attributes this fact to a cause the existence of which is not commonly recognized. It is here quite a matter of indifference whether such movements are, according to the tenets of spiritualism, attributable to the machinations of spirits, or whether they are due, as the psychists contend, to special psychical powers inherent in the medium. When A concentrates his thoughts upon a fixed subject, and B unconsciously follows the same strain of thought, the occultist looks upon this manifestation as a reflex of A's influence over B's mind. The community at large does not recognize this influence, but assumes, rather, that B arrived at his thoughts in a more natural manner- for instance, by pre-concerted action, or by whispered communications, or by other obvious means, acquainting B with the thoughts of A, or else by sheer coincidence.

An American investigator has, e.g, found that the majority of people have a decided preference for certain numbers, and, strange to say, in psychical experiments these very numbers occur more frequently than any others. Now, if A and B happen to accidentally give preference to the same favorite numbers, it will not appear strange that both will arrive at the same result more frequently than the theories of probability would seem to warrant. One thing seems to be quite clear- that all occult manifestations have one thing in common, namely, that they emanate from a source which is not generally recognized to exist, whether this be found in the phenomenon itself, as in the case of the fakir, or in its cause, as in table-rapping and furniture-moving, or in the relations existing between the manifestations themselves and their causes, as in transference of thought, or telepathy.

But occult phenomena have also one other thing in common- viz., the circumstance that their causative element is, according to occultism, to be found in psychical- i.e., in personal forces. For instance, science today teaches us that a rain of sand or ashes or frogs is a phenomenon due to meteorological causes, but by no means resulting from personal influences. If, however, such a phenomenon should be proclaimed, as of yore, to be the manifestation of a spirit world, it would at once come under the range of occultism.

Occult phenomena have, therefore, two things in common- first, that they originate from a cause not generally understood or recognized; and, secondly, that this cause is to be found in some psychical being. From this a close relationship between Christian Science and occultism will at once become apparent. In the first place, no one will deny that in Christian Science many things happen which are in direct opposition ta common experience; for instance, cancer may be cured by concentrating one's thoughts upon the fact that God does not desire sin, but disease- e.g., cancer- is the consequence of sin, therefore God will heal it. On the other hand, certain phenomena are referred by Christian Science to the direct influence of psychical beings other than God Himself. Mrs. Eddy and her followers lay special stress upon the circumstance that the surroundings exercise a particular influence upon the cure- nay, that the cure chiefly depends upon the psychical influence of some individual capable of sufficient concentration of mind over another individual. Hence it follows that self-cure is absolutely excluded, but that the medium of a second person- i.e, the Christian Scientist- is indispensable.

This interference of a second person strongly suggests animal magnetism, and, in fact, Christian Science openly speaks of 'currents' of which one hears so much in animal magnetism and spiritualistic seances. But other miracle-workers besides Mrs. Eddy have claimed this magnetic element, and it has been discussed more than once. In the beginning of the nineteenth century Prince Hohenlohe, a Catholic priest, created quite a sensation in this direction- viz., in 1821 in Bavaria- and elsewhere during subsequent years. The adherents of animal magnetism looked upon him as a man possessed of exceptional powers, whilst others attributed the wonderful cures he accomplished to the direct influence of religious belief.

But there are other relations existing between occultism and Christian Science. Treatment from a distance infallibly suggests telepathy. That Christian Science is the direct intermediary between the patient and God is another proof of its intimate affinity to spiritualism, for in both the manifestations are dependent upon the interference of a medium. Under these circumstances it will not appear strange that many followers of Christian Science are also devotees of spiritualism and occultism- in fact, many a Christian Science healer enjoys the fame of being a noted medium.

Even where an apparent distinction between Scientist, spiritualist, and occultist is claimed, it does not in reality exist, for scientism and occultism converge in the same focus. Much depends on the surroundings and circumstances whether the healer gravitates more to occultism or to spiritualism. It matters little that Mrs. Eddy, in her work on 'Christian Science' inveighs against occultism and animal magnetism. This does not change the fact, nor is it in the least affected by the disclaimers of some of her followers. The connection is too evident, and that is the main point. I have in the foregoing discussion attempted to make plain the relations in which Christian Science stands to medicine and occultism. I have abstained from personal attacks and treated the subject in the abstract. My researches were made both in America and in Berlin, and my information is gained not only from persons who have been treated by Christian Scientists, but also from Christian Science healers themselves, who, I must admit, gave it ungrudgingly.

I have purposely not touched upon the point whether these healers- Mrs. Eddy herself included- are actuated by good faith or not, for so far as the interests of the public are concerned this carries but little weight. The fact that the healers take money for their attendance does, in my opinion, in no way impeach their *bona fides* as some seem to think; for no man can make himself independent of social conditions, and money is necessary for one's maintenance. The same might be said of spiritualistic media, although even many believers fight shy of those who demand payment. (Perhaps the medium belonging to 'society' who gives stances without pay is, after all, the more dangerous of the two, since the very suspicion that Mrs. X could be guilty of swindling or deception would produce indignation, and scientific tests and research are rendered much more difficult under these circumstances than in the case of a paid medium.)

I think this standpoint is false, for material interests are not always the necessary motives for swindling; often enough the pleasures derived from deception, or ambition, or vanity are sufficiently strong incentives. If Christian Science is a peril, the fact that the healers are personally honest cannot affect the truth. If we approach the matter from the practical side of the question, as to whether Christian Science can really benefit a patient, I think it cannot be denied that under given circumstances it may be of use- i.e. in cases where psychical treatment is indicated.

So far as the physician is concerned, the doubtful and critical element of treatment by Christian Science is not so much to be found in what it accomplishes, but in what it omits. This, however, may be said of every quack treatment. Certain it is that cancer, for instance, may become incurable if timely operation is delayed. Appendicitis, like other suppurations, may lead to the gravest complications unless it is taken in hand promptly and by the proper authority. No matter how skeptically medical skill and science may be regarded, there are doubtless many cases in which neglect and delay will aggravate the disease and surely bring about a fatal issue. For which reason it behooves the medical profession to stigmatize as dangerous any method by which diseases are treated without preceding proper diagnosis, no matter whether it is a Kneipp cure, or treatment by animal magnetism, or Christian Science. Of course, the Christian Scientists claim that the patients who come to them for treatment would not in any case undergo an operation. Even granted, this would only prove that in such a case the false hope of a cure by other than the legitimate means was raised in the mind of the patient, though not necessarily by this or that particular faith-healer. But if the Christian Scientists deny the possibility of a curable disease becoming incurable during the time of treatment by Christian Science- that cancer, for instance, could only be improved thereby, and that curable affections could, at any rate, not turn into incurable diseases- further discussion must come to an end in the face of such ignorance and denseness. To arrive at an agreement with such people is as impossible as a discussion between two foreigners ignorant of each other's language.

Christian Science belongs to the category of psychical epidemics, which are bound to come among us now and then. Often they disappear as mysteriously and rapidly as they come, but sometimes they linger a long time. To the arguments of reason they do not yield, and even the law seems to be impotent in checking their career. How difficult it is to combat these evils may be evident from an incident which came recently under my observation in Berlin. When the flower-medium, Mrs. Rothe, was arrested by the police for swindling and deception, that group of spiritualists who frequented her stances denied the charges made by the police authorities against her. They seriously declared that, although Mrs. Rothe purchased with money the flowers used at her stances, these self-same flowers were bought whilst in a materialized condition; but Mrs. Rothe dematerialized the flowers, and employed them in that condition for her functions.

But when Mrs. Rothe came into physical contact with the detective who effected her arrest, the flowers suddenly became materialized again, and in this manner the poor woman innocently came under the suspicion of being a fraud and an impostor. All this goes to show that the law cannot adequately deal with these excrescences, although it may often act as a beneficent aid in combating them. The present sociological conditions prevailing in Germany as well as in other civilized countries undoubtedly offer a fertile ground for this psychical epidemic.

To the impartial observer of occultism this is quite obvious. When in the latter part of the eighties I began to make a closer study of this subject, I could trace, for instance, in Berlin only one society of occultists. It was called 'Verein Psyche,' and held its meetings every Friday evening at the 'Prelat.' Now the 'Event of the Day' contain daily announcements of one or more such meetings. There are the Theosophic Society, Berlin Branch; the Christian Theosophic Society; the Scientific Union Sphinx; the Spiritualistic Lodge, 'Psyche of Truth'; the Spiritualistic Club Empor; the Spiritualistic Union Sunlight; the Spiritualistic Union Eos z. E. the Magnetic Society.

Instructive, however, is the fact that, as a rule, but little love is lost between these various societies. Each claims to be the only one that is founded on the genuine scientific principles of occultism, and therefore disparages the merits of the others in due proportion. It would be a fallacy to assume that the followers of occultism and spiritualism are solely recruited from degenerates and imbeciles. Many of their members are highly endowed with mental gifts. Anyone who has attended their discussions will be impressed with this truth. Yet whatever passes at these meetings under the pretense of science or scientific research is a clear proof that these people know little or nothing of the true aims of science, and that they are quite incapable of grasping and appreciating the labors and difficulties encountered in genuine scientific research. Far be it from me to claim for science the right to belittle or repudiate the efforts of the layman. But, on the other hand, I cannot admit that every uneducated or half-witted individual who dabbles in scientific matters has the right to call himself a man of science on the ground that many valuable discoveries in the field of science have been made by laymen. And conceit, forsooth, is as a rule the chief virtue which adorns the spiritualist.

It will also be found that many of these people are easily impressed by anything which deviates from the normal rule, and thus it may not be a mere accident when we discover that many spiritualists are also strong believers in Dr. Jaeger's sanitary wool theory, are enthusiastic homoeopaths or strict vegetarians, are sworn enemies of the regular school of medicine, and- who can tell?- perhaps, also, inveterate Baconites. The capable men among them- whom no one would suspect of being spiritualists- are generally known to the initiated only, for they do not parade their connection in public. Perhaps this occultistic, spiritualistic, and scientistic movement is but the reaction of that extreme materialism which was rampant in the sixties of the last century.

Extremes often converge. If we may judge by signs, well, then, the modern occultist is as arrogant and presumptuous as the materialist was of old, who blatantly undertook to explain psychical processes by the simple application of a few catchwords or stock phrases. It would be a mistake to stigmatize everything said or assumed by occultism as sheer nonsense, unworthy of test or research. On the contrary, the man who does not pass by these questions without giving them due notice renders a great service to enlightenment. But the research must be seriously carried out on behalf of science and in truly scientific fashion. Of course, this cannot be done by men who, as soon as they hear the creaking of a piece of furniture, immediately jump to the conclusion that some restless spirit of another world wishes to make a communication. The regulations

36

of spiritualism render all rational tests futile, since they rigidly exclude and prevent all means of precaution under the plea that these act only as a perturbing element in the very experiments by which, strange to say, the spiritualist seeks to convince.

For many years I have made occultistic phenomena my particular study. I have explored telepathy, cures from a distance, animal magnetism, table-moving, spirit rapping, materializations, and so-called fire-media. But I can conscientiously state that I have never come across a single phenomenon which was not open to explanation by those forces known to reputable science. I never found it necessary to call to my aid the hypothesis of spirit intervention or of mysterious psychical forces to explain such manifestations as came under my notice.

All my tests were carried out on the basis of genuine scientific principles. But I have been often thwarted in my object, because the conditions I imposed were not adhered to, although I had been solemnly assured that they should be honored. This is one of the chief tricks of the spiritualistic medium. Test-experiments, though promised, are invariably shirked. The audience is assured that the experiments are carried out under strict observance of all conditions and demands made by science, whilst practically this is never done. A typical example is the case of Mrs. Rothe, about whom Erich Bohn wrote a comprehensive treatise in igoi. He proposed to her repeatedly several committees for the proper examination into her manifestations (the committee in Berlin was to consist of Dr. Dessoir and myself)- But Mrs. Rothe would have none of these committees. And yet in spite of this her followers declared that every means of precaution was adopted to preclude even the possibility of fraud.

Practically no tests, such as would satisfy science, were

ever instituted at Mrs. Rothe's seances. Wherever else they were applied, the fraud was unerringly laid bare. The common subterfuge of the spiritualists, of course, is that the very presence of a skeptical person and the observance of strict conditions frustrate the manifestations of the spirit world. But if this be the case, and the conditions demanded by science cannot be fulfilled, then it is wrong to allege that scientific tests have been made either on behalf of spiritualism or occultism or Christian Science.

The theologians emphatically deny that any of these movements have root in the Christian doctrine. I maintain, with, I flatter myself, the universal support of all scientific men, that none of them, especially not Christian Science, are fathered by science.

THE END